BIG-ASS SALADS

31 Easy Recipes for Your Healthy Month

Duc Vuong, M.D.

ISBN-13: 978-0692987001

ISBN-10: 0692987002

Published by HappyStance Publishing. Interior formatting and cover design by Tony Loton of LOTONtech Limited, www.lotontech.com.

 The information and recipes contained within the "Big-Ass Salads" book are based on extensive research conducted by the author. The sources used for the research are credible and authentic to the best of our knowledge. The nutrition advices are designed for an average healthy man and woman who have no health problems. Before using this book, be sure to consult a doctor. In no event shall the author be liable for any direct, indirect, incidental, punitive, or consequential damages of any kind whatsoever with respect to the service, the materials and the products contained within. This book is not a substitute for professional nutrition or health advice.

For My Patients,

who inspire me every day with their courage.

Contents

Introduction

I am a huge salad fan! And what is there not to love? These easy to make, well-balanced meals made me create this book and share some of my favorite recipes with you. I have one salad as the main meal a day. **I teach my patients to try and eat a 50% raw diet.**

While achieving this percentage might seem difficult for most people, it's quite simple. Here's how:

1) Have a green smoothie for breakfast: A green smoothie consists of some greens (such as spinach or kale), some fresh or frozen fruit (like banana or frozen berries), and a liquid base (like water, soy milk, or almond milk.) For more smoothie recipes, please check out my book, Healthy Green Smoothies: 50 Easy Recipes That Will Change Your Life. It's available on Amazon.com.

2) Have one Big-Ass Salad a day as your main meal: You can add beans, tofu, fish, grilled shrimp, or even meat to complete the meal. But make sure that the salad is the main star and not just the sidekick.

If you follow these two simple rules you should have a diet that is approximately 66% raw.

This book will help you solve the everyday problem of healthy eating and overcome the fear of complicated recipes. I have minimized the cooking, baking, and frying. Go fresh and get on with making some healthy changes to repair a damage that processed food has done to your body.

A diet full of fresh fruits, leafy greens, vegetables, beans, whole grains like cooked quinoa, fish, and seafood is one of the healthiest diets in the world, especially when combined with healthy fats from olive oil, nuts, and seeds. The best part is that after just a couple of days, you will begin to feel the health benefits. Our bodies have a powerful ability to heal in a way that we are just beginning to discover. Toss a bunch of leafy greens, fresh veggies, add some healthy, Omega-3 rich olive oil, sprinkle with some herbs for extra flavor and create a perfect meal at home or on the go.

We all make our own choices but your choice to pick up this book is a good one for your overall health. Enjoy the recipes and leave me your comments and reviews on Amazon. I always like to hear from readers!

1. Frisee Salad with a Champagne Vinaigrette

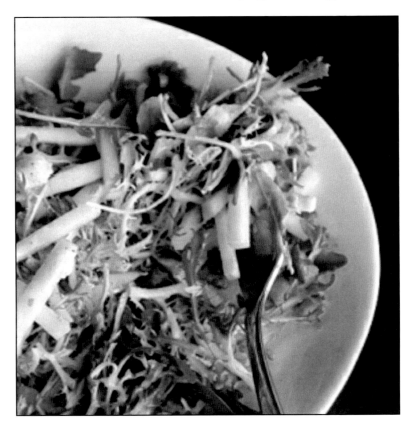

Looking for a great starter salad? This healthy frisee mix, with a gentle touch of champagne vinaigrette, is my favorite, easy to follow salad formula. A few simple ingredients make this salad extremely quick to make, which is great for when you're in a hurry. And the best thing about it – it tastes perfect every time!

Ingredients:

- 1 pound frisee, trimmed and roughly torn
- 1 handful of walnuts
- 1 small honeycrisp apple
- ¼ cup of champagne vinegar
- 3 tsp of Dijon mustard
- ½ cup of olive oil
- ¼ tsp of salt
- Pinch of ground, black pepper

Preparation:

Combine champagne vinegar, Dijon mustard, olive oil, salt, and pepper in a blender. Blend well to combine. Set aside.

Trim and roughly torn the frisee in a bowl. Slice the apple into thin matchsticks. Combine with frisee, add about a handful of walnuts and a generous drizzle of the vinaigrette. Toss well to combine. Serve cold.

2. Spring Strawberry Salad

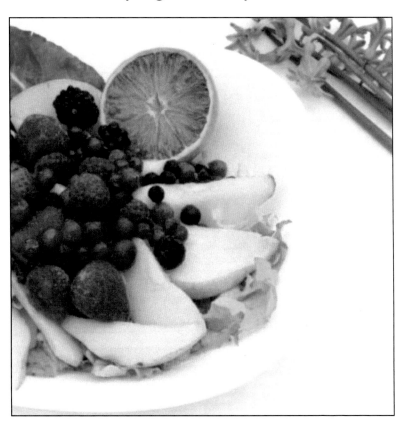

Spring strawberry salad is a classic snack that works for every occasion. A delicious combination of wild berries with the ultimate refreshing taste of the orange juice and sweet nutmeg is a perfect meal that you can make in less than ten minutes. Enjoy this salad without the fear of gaining weight. The only thing you can gain with this salad are the numerous amounts of vitamins and minerals.

Ingredients:

- 1 cup of mixed fresh berries
- 5-6 medium-sized strawberries
- ½ pear, sliced
- 2oz fresh spinach
- ¼ cup fresh orange juice
- 1 tsp of sugar
- ¼ tsp of nutmeg

Preparation:

In a small bowl, combine the fresh orange juice with sugar and nutmeg. Mix well with a fork. Add mixed berries to bowl and gently combine.

Wash and gently rinse the spinach. Pat dry with paper towels. Place on a serving plate.

Slice pear and make a second layer on your plate. Spoon on mixed berries. Drizzle orange juice dressing. Top with the fresh strawberries. Serve cold.

A great tip is to leave it in the freezer for ten minutes before serving.

3. Energy Boost Lunch Pack

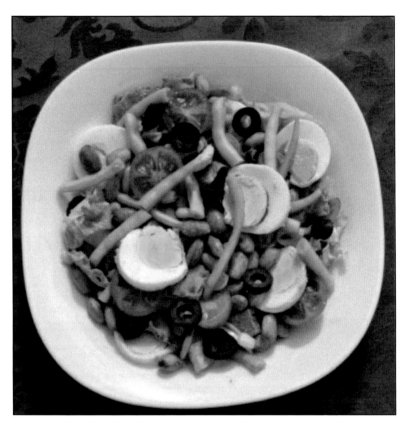

Rushed for lunch? Go classic and chunky, but hold the mayo! Perfectly hard-boiled eggs are thinly sliced then sprinkled with a simple vinaigrette and combined with salty olives, fiber-packed beans, and vitamin C abundant cherry tomatoes.

Ingredients:

- 1 boiled egg
- 1 cup of lettuce, finely chopped
- ½ cup of green beans, cooked
- ½ cup kidney beans, cooked
- 4 cherry tomatoes, halved
- Few black olives, sliced
- 3 tbsp of extra virgin olive oil
- ½ tsp of salt
- 1 tbsp of fresh lemon juice

Preparation:

To boil the egg, gently place the egg into a pot with just enough water to cover it. Bring to a boil and cook for another 8 minutes. You can use a kitchen timer. After 8 minutes, drain the water and place the egg under the cold water. Peel and slice.

Meanwhile, combine the other ingredients in a large bowl. Add the olive oil, fresh lemon juice, and salt. Toss well to combine. Top with sliced eggs and serve.

4. Kiwi Berry Salad

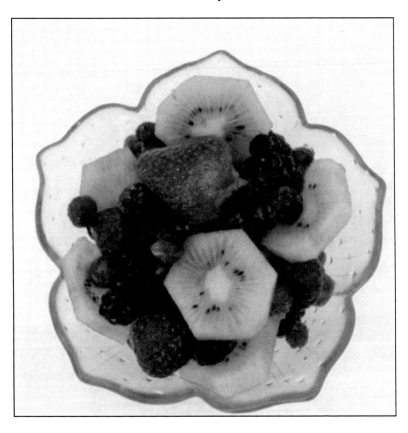

It's amazing how only a few ingredients with a drizzle of honey with a splash of lemon can taste so sensational! Kiwifruit is an excellent source of vitamin C and vitamin K and will lighten up your everyday snack. Vibrant colors and flavors make this simple fruit salad an exceptional refreshing spring combination. Try it for breakfast.

Ingredients:

- 1 kiwi, peeled and sliced
- 1 cup of mixed berries
- 1 tbsp of honey
- ¼ cup of fresh lime juice

Preparation:

Combine the honey with fresh lime juice. Mix well with a fork and pour in a bowl. Toss with the fruit and leave in the refrigerator for about 20 minutes before serving.

5. Curly Kale with Fresh Apple Juice Dressing

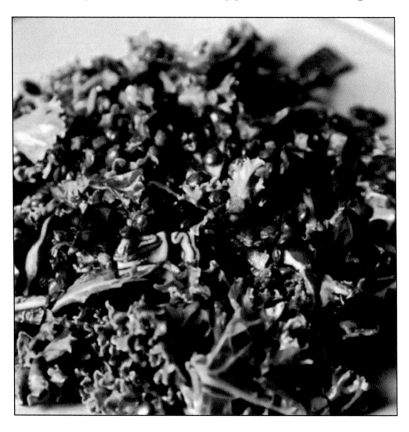

This tasty kale salad with a lentil twist is a perfect option for both a fancy brunch or a quiet dinner at home. Apple juice dressing elevates these lively flavors into a heavenly harmonious realm. Use leftover lentils for a faster preparation.

Ingredients (salad):

- A bunch of curly kale, roughly chopped
- 1 cup of red cabbage, thinly shredded
- ½ cup of cooked red lentils

Ingredients (dressing):

- ¼ cup of olive oil
- ¼ cup of freshly squeezed apple juice
- 1 tsp of apple cider vinegar
- 2 tbsp of freshly squeezed lemon juice
- ½ tsp of salt 2 tsp of yellow mustard

Preparation:

Whisk together the dressing ingredients in a small bowl. Keep in the refrigerator before serving.

Meanwhile, cook the lentils. For ½ cup of lentils, you will need 1 ½ cup of water as the lentils will double in size. Cook for about 15 minutes, or until the lentils have softened. Remove from the heat and drain. Cool to room temp.

Combine the lentils with roughly chopped kale and thinly shredded red cabbage. Mix well and serve with apple juice dressing. Toss to combine.

6. Simple Spring Salad

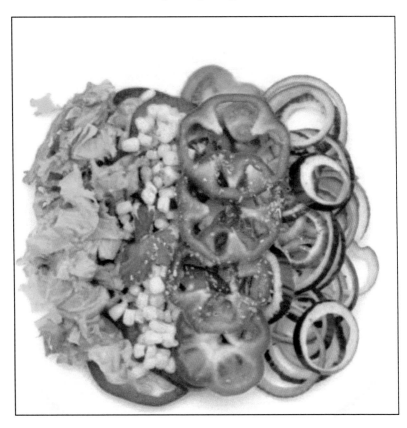

Spring is the perfect time to play with different colors and aromas. This visually-stunning recipe uses naturally vibrant hues to paint a perfect masterpiece on your plate. Any readily available vegetable can be a part of your color palette. Sprinkle some dry rosemary to give it a spring kick.

Ingredients:

- ½ cup of Romaine lettuce, finely chopped
- ½ cup of sweet raw corn (about 1 raw corn cob)
- 1 red bell pepper, sliced
- ½ green bell pepper, sliced
- 5 cherry tomatoes, halved
- ½ red onion, peeled and sliced
- 1 tsp of dry rosemary, crushed
- Fresh lime juice
- Salt and Pepper to taste

Preparation:

Wash and cut the bell peppers in half. Remove the seeds and the pulp. Cut into thin slices.

Peel and slice the onion. If desired, soak the onion rings in warm water for 10 minutes to cut the rawness.

Remove the husk and silk off the corn cob. Using a sharp knife, cut the kernels off the cob. With the blunt side of the blade, scrape the cob to get out the corn milk.

Use a big serving platter and arrange the vegetables. You can play with some colors, or even add some ingredients you like. Sprinkle with some rosemary, fresh lime juice, and the corn milk. Salt and pepper to taste. Serve immediately.

7. Student Medley Mix

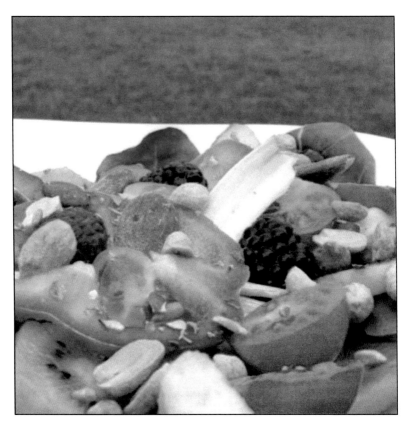

This smorgasbord of ingredients is reminiscent of a college pool party—everybody in! Clear out the pantry for this one. The tart sweetness of blackberries compliments the flavor of leafy greens, like a keg in a dorm room. Fresh kiwifruit slices provide the antioxidant Vitamin C. Mixed nuts add a tasty crunch for a nice bite.

Ingredients (salad):

- ½ pear sliced
- 1 kiwi, peeled and sliced
- Few cherry tomatoes, halved
- ½ cup of wild berries
- ½ cup of nut mix
- ½ green bell pepper, sliced

Ingredients (dressing):

- 2 tbsp of honey
- ¼ cup of fresh lime juice
- 1 tsp of mustard

Preparation:

Whisk fresh lime juice, mustard and honey with a fork. In a large bowl, combine the vegetables and add the dressing. Toss well to combine.

8. Grilled Shrimp Skewers with Lemon-Chili Dressing

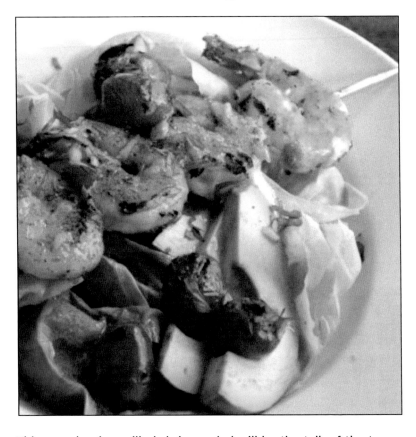

This eye-pleasing grilled shrimp salad will be the talk of the town when you make it. You can easily combine any vegetables you like, and the shrimps will transform that salad mixture into a feast fit for a king and queen.

Ingredients (grilled shrimps and tomatoes):

- 5 large shrimp (per person), peeled and deveined
- 8 grape tomatoes (per person)
- 2 skewers, soaked in water

Ingredients (marinade):

- olive oil, enough to make a runny paste

- 2 garlic cloves, crushed
- 1 tsp of fresh cilantro, minced
- ½ tsp of turmeric powder
- Salt and pepper to taste

Ingredients (salad):

- ½ head butter lettuce, roughly chopped
- ½ avocado, sliced

Ingredients (lemon-chili dressing):

- ¼ cup of freshly squeezed lemon juice
- ¼ cup of extra virgin olive oil
- 1 tsp of dijon mustard
- ¼ tsp of chili powder
- ½ tsp of cumin, ground
- 1 tbsp of scallions, minced
- ¼ tsp of sea salt

Preparation:

For the marinade, mix together three tablespoons of olive oil, crushed garlic, fresh cilantro, turmeric powder, salt, and pepper. Stir until completely combined.

Skewer your shrimps and tomatoes and spread the marinade over it using a kitchen brush. Let skewers sit for 30 minutes.

Preheat an electric grill over a high temperature. In a pinch, you can also use a saute pan. On lazy Sundays, you can fire up the grill.

Grill the skewers for about 3 minutes on each side. Remove from the grill and set aside.

Combine the lemon-chili dressing ingredients in a small bowl. Place the butter lettuce and avocado on a plate. Drizzle with the lemon-chili dressing. Top with the shrimp and tomato skewers.

9. Classic Warm Italian Asparagus Salad

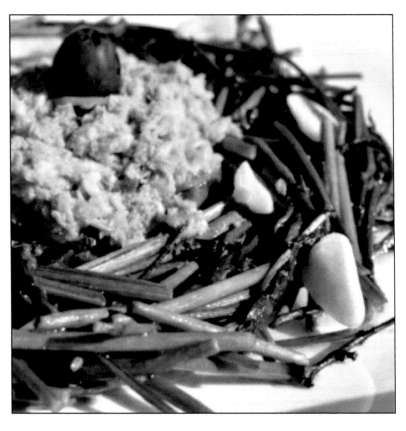

Lightly sauteed asparagus with its nutty flavor is the base of this healthy salad. Combined with garlic and topped with the ubiquitous tuna, this salad becomes the rescue for a lunchtime executive on the go. Serve this warm salad immediately.

Ingredients:

- ½ pound of fresh asparagus
- 3 tbsp of tuna, without oil. You can substitute black beans instead.
- 2 cloves of garlic
- Your favorite olives
- 2 tbsp of vegetable oil, for frying
- 3 tbsp of extra virgin olive oil
- Salt to taste

Preparation:

Clean and cut the asparagus into 2 inch long strips. Heat up 2 tbsp of vegetable oil over a medium-high temperature. Add asparagus and stir-fry for several minutes. Remove from the heat and use some kitchen paper to soak the excess oil. Transfer to a serving platter and top with tuna. Season with salt and olive oil. Decorate with some black olives.

10. Roasted Beet, Gala Apple and Spinach Salad

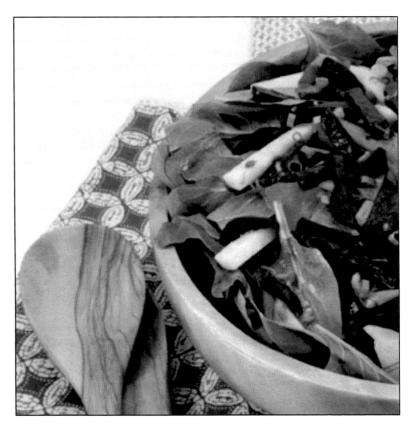

This beautiful combination is hearty enough to be a staple at Thanksgiving. If your childhood memories of beets involve a can opener, then your culinary taste buds are about to elevate. Roasting beets is simply, in my opinion, the best way to prepare beets. The crisp apple compliments the tender beets perfectly in this simple yet tasty recipe. Save the beet greens for another salad.

Ingredients (salad):

- 2 large beets, roasted and sliced
- 2 cups of spinach, trimmed
- 2 spring onions, finely chopped
- 1 gala apple

Ingredients (dressing):

- ¼ cup of olive oil
- 2 tbsp of fresh lime juice
- 1 tbsp of granulated sugar
- 1 garlic clove, crushed
- 1 tsp of apple cider
- ¼ tsp of pepper
- ¼ tsp of salt

Preparation:

Preheat the oven to 375 degrees. Trim the green tops off the beets. Save the greens for another salad.

Poke several holes in the beets with a fork. Wrap them tightly in aluminum foil. Roast them in the oven for about 60 minutes or until tender. Remove the skin and slice. Transfer to a bowl.

Combine olive oil, vinegar, cider, salt, pepper, and sugar. Pour over beet slices and toss to coat. Let stand for at least 30 minutes.

Wash and pat dry the apple. Slice into thin strips and combine with beet slices, spring onions, and spinach. Add crushed garlic and mix well. Serve.

11. Warm Beet Greens and Kale with Garlic Dressing

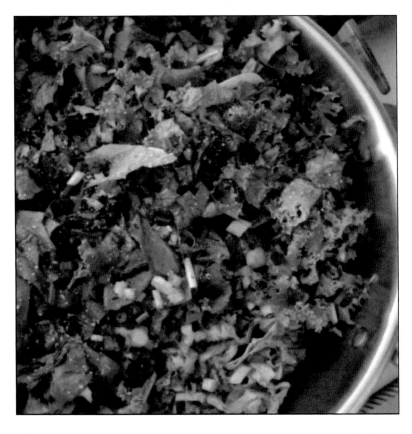

Did you know that you can use beet greens as a salad? Beet greens are an excellent source of iron, providing 15%of the daily recommended amount in just one cup of serving. When you combine it with kale and spring onions, you get a highly nutritious meal.

Ingredients (salad):

- 1 cup of beet greens, rinsed and chopped
- 2 cups of kale, rinsed and chopped
- 2 spring onions, finely chopped

Ingredients (dressing):

- 2 garlic cloves, crushed
- 3 tbsp of cilantro, finely chopped
- 1 orange
- ¼ cup of raw cashews
- ¼ cup of olive oil
- A pinch of salt

Preparation:

Combine the dressing ingredients in a food processor and mix well until creamy mixture. Set aside.

Place the beet greens in a saucepan and pour enough water to cover. Bring it to a boil and cook for a couple of minutes. Remove from the heat and drain. Cool for a while and transfer to a bowl. Add chopped kale and spring onion, pour the dressing over the salad and toss well to combine.

12. Hot Mexican Wraps

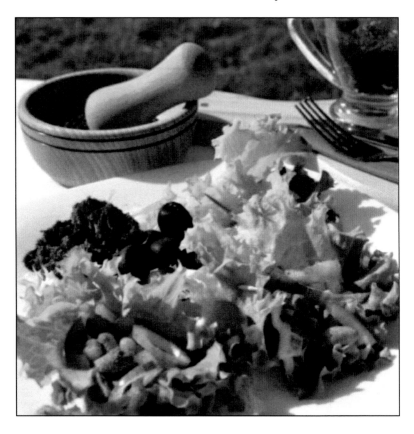

Everybody loves hot Mexican wraps that are bursting with flavor. But, let's try a healthier version of this world famous dish. Replace the processed flour tortillas with crispy lettuce; spread the protein-rich beans, fresh vegetables and sprinkle with spicy chilly. I promise you won't be able to keep your hands off this fabulous snack.

Ingredients:

- 3 large lettuce leaves
- ¼ cup of kidney beans, cooked
- ½ tomato, chopped
- ¼ cup of sweet corn
- ½ red onion, peeled and sliced
- 1 tsp of ground chili pepper
- Salt to taste
- Your favorite hot sauce
- ½ tsp of apple cider vinegar

Preparation:

In a bowl, combine the kidney beans with tomato, sweet corn, and red onion slices. Season with ground chili pepper, apple cider vinegar, hot sauce, and some salt to taste.

Place 2 tbsp of this mixture over each lettuce leaf. Wrap and secure with toothpicks. Serve with fresh Mexican salsa.

13. Two Peas in a Pod Salad

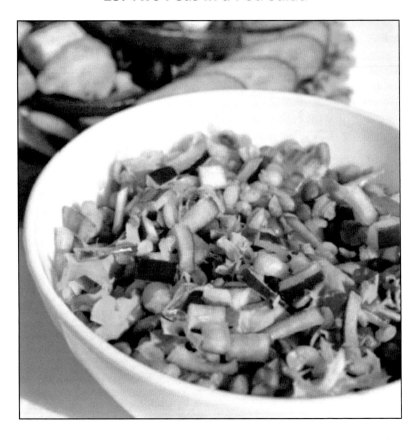

Place all the ingredients in a bowl and mix well. Before serving add three tablespoons of cherry vinaigrette and toss to coat. In this recipe, lentils and chickpeas are like best friends enjoying a sunny day in a hammock. That is until sharp onion tries to muscle in on the act. Ultimately, the three manage to get along in a harmonious union, which reminds me of the old television show, Three's Company.

Ingredients:

- ½ cup of cooked lentils
- ½ cup of cooked chickpeas
- ½ red onion, finely chopped
- 1 cup of lettuce, finely chopped
- 3 tbsp of cherry vinaigrette

Preparation:

Place all ingredients in a bowl and mix well. Before serving add two tablespoons of cherry vinaigrette and toss to coat.

14. Rainbow Swiss Chard with Toasted Pine Nuts

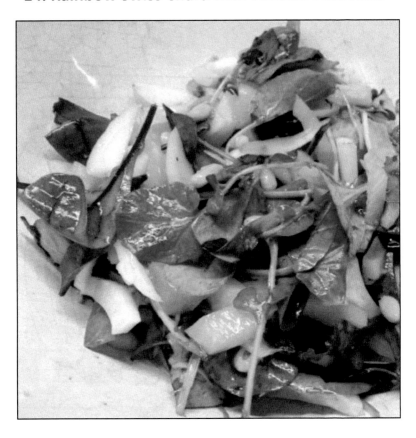

Swiss chard is definitely one of my favorite ingredients in salads. Its tender flavor is not the only reason why these leafy greens are so popular. Swiss chard is loaded with vitamin K, vitamin A, vitamin C, magnesium, copper, manganese, potassium, vitamin E, and iron. A drizzle of walnut oil in this salad will protect your heart and blood vessels. But despite the health benefits, it's the mystery and elegance of the name "Swiss chard" that tugs at my heartstrings. Impress even the harshest food critic will this offering.

Ingredients:

- A handful of fresh Rainbow Swiss chard
- 1 medium-sized yellow bell pepper, sliced
- 1 small green apple, chopped
- ¼ cup of pine nuts, lightly toasted
- ¼ of a raw fennel bulb, chopped into bite-sized pieces
- 2 tbsp of walnut oil
- 2 tbsp of sherry vinegar
- Salt, to taste
- Pepper, to taste

Preparation:

Combine the vegetables in a large bowl. Add apple slices and pine nuts. Drizzle with the sherry vinegar and walnut oil. Season with salt and pepper and toss to combine.

15. Mesclun Salad with Mussels

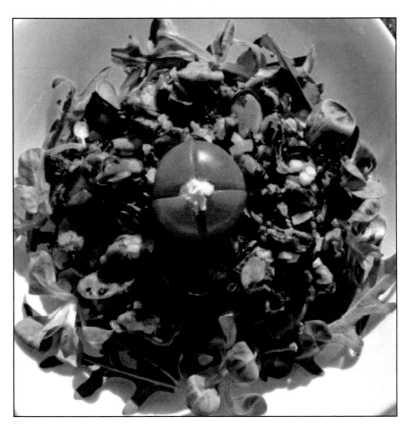

The original Mesclun salad recipe comes from Provence, France. It is a fresh and healthy mix of arugula, chervil, endive and leafy lettuces. The vinaigrette is the salty-sour flavor people love so much. However, these greens can do a little more than that. The exciting combination of fresh mussels with a touch of garlic gives the classic Mesclun a bit of vibrant, Italian flavor. The leafy part supplies plenty of "foliage vitamin" - folate, while the mussels provide you with the vitamin A, B-vitamins, phosphorus, zinc, manganese, and omega-3 fatty acids. You can dress it up with ripe tomatoes or even black olives.

Ingredients:

- 2 pounds of fresh mussels, debearded
- 1 large onion, peeled and finely chopped
- ¼ cup of vegetable stock (or water)
- 3 cloves of garlic, crushed
- 5 tbsp of olive oil
- ¼ cup of fresh parsley, finely chopped
- 1 tbsp of rosemary, finely chopped
- ½ cup of arugula leaves
- 1 medium cherry tomato, for decoration
- Salt to taste

Preparation:

Rinse and drain the mussels. Set aside.

Heat up 2 tbsp of olive oil over medium-high temperature in a pan. Peel and finely chop the onion. Reduce the heat to medium temperature and add the chopped onion. Saute for several minutes, until tender. Now add the mussels and finely chopped parsley. Add some salt. Add vegetable stock.

Cover tightly with lid and cook for about 8 minutes, shaking the skillet regularly. When the mussels have opened, add garlic, chopped rosemary and mix well again.

In a large bowl, combine the mussels with arugula. Add the remaining oil, sprinkle with some salt, and decorate with one cherry tomato. Serve immediately.

16. Geeky Greek Chicken Salad

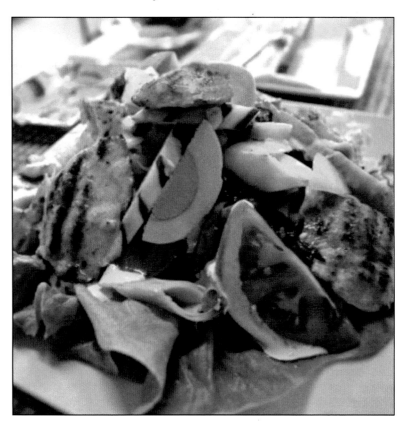

This chicken salad recipe with a touch of geeky Greek-style is the most cooking we will do in this book. Don't fret—you can use the boiled eggs and cooked chicken for other dishes. Create multiple flavor combinations simply by adding some of your favorite ingredients.

Ingredients:

- 1 boiled egg ripe tomato, sliced
- Romaine lettuce leaves, rinsed
- ½ cup of red cabbage, thinly sliced
- 1 cucumber, sliced
- ½ piece of chicken breast, boneless and skinless
- Few black olives
- 2 tbsp of Greek olive oil
- 1 tbsp of plain Greek yogurt
- 1 tbsp of fresh lemon juice
- Sea salt to taste

Preparation:

Thinly slice the red cabbage. Transfer to bowl. Sprinkle some salt and let it stand for about zo minutes. Squeeze out any water that has extracted from the cabbage. Sprinkle the lemon juice all over it.

Meanwhile, put the eggs into a pot of boiling water. Be very gentle while doing this to avoid accidentally cracking the eggs. One useful tip to prepare the perfect boiled eggs is to add 1 tbsp of baking soda into the boiling water. This will make a peeling process much easier. Boil the eggs for 8 minutes. After 8 minutes, drain the water and place the eggs under cold water for a few minutes. Peel and slice the eggs.

Wash and pat dry the chicken. Season with salt and pepper. Preheat a nonstick pan and add the chicken breast. The trick is to add small amounts of water (1-2 tbsp) as often as needed. Cook the chicken breast for about 8-6 minutes per side, depending on thickness. Remove from the pan and allow it to rest.

Combine the vegetables in a large bowl, add eggs, chicken breast and top with some Greek yogurt. Sprinkle some more salt and add the olive oil. Toss well to combine and serve immediately.

17. Edamame Superfood Salad

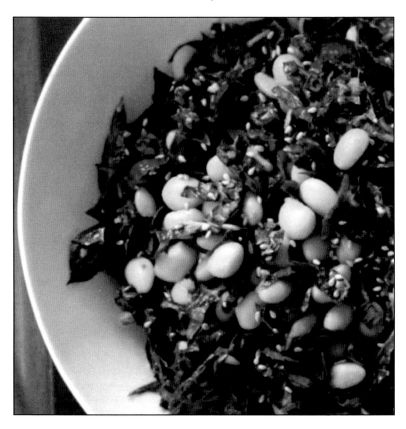

Edamame is truly a star legume. Sure, edamame is just a fancy word for soybeans, but oh, isn't it more fun to say ED-uh-MOMmy? This superfood is packed with fiber, protein, vitamins, and minerals. Combined with kale and sesame oil, it creates one tasty super salad.

Ingredients:

- 2 cups kale, thinly sliced
- ½ cup of boiled edamame
- 2 tbsp of fresh lemon juice
- 1 tbsp of sesame seeds
- 2 tbsp of sesame oil
- 2 tbsp of agave nectar
- 2 garlic cloves, crushed
- A pinch of salt

Preparation:

Briefly boil the edamame (about 3-4 minutes will be enough). If fresh edamame is not available, then frozen edamame can often be found in the frozen foods aisle.

Add two cups of kale in a large bowl and mix with edamame. Combine with lemon juice, sesame oil, agave nectar, crushed garlic, and salt. Mix well until wilted. Serve.

18. Orange Sunshine Salad

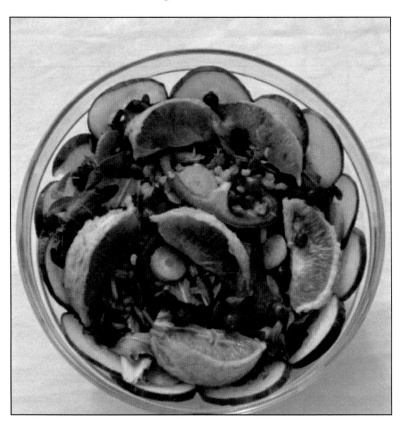

I like this salad because it is just a really fabulous, sunshiny twist on boring salads. Topped with sweet oranges and tiny gooseberries, this salad is something new and unexpected. But when you scratch under the surface, you will find a real gold mine of nutrition. Definitely worth trying.

Ingredients (salad):

- ½ cup of cooked lentils
- ½ cup of finely chopped argula
- ½ cucumber, sliced
- ½ orange, peeled and sectioned
- ½ carrot, sliced
- ½ green bell pepper, sliced
- ¼ cup of fresh gooseberries

Ingredients (Balsamic-Dijon vinaigrette):

- 1 tsp of balsamic vinegar
- 1 tbs of dijon mustard
- ¼ cup of olive oil
- ½ tsp of ground red pepper
- ¼ tsp of salt

Preparation:

Combine the vegetables in a large bowl. Add lentils and mix well. Set aside.

In a smaller bowl, shake together the balsamic vinegar, dijon mustard, olive oil, salt, and red pepper. Pour the vinaigrette over the vegetables and mix well. Top with orange and gooseberries.

19. Seafood Skewers

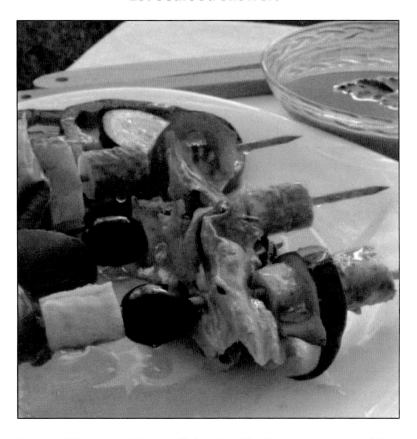

Bored with usual BBQ food? Maybe it's time to try something new. These healthy kabobs are a nice change. It is amazing how easily you can turn something so simple into true satisfaction. They feature crispy cucumber, soft, ripe tomatoes and delicious olives. Tossed with fresh lime juice, extra virgin olive oil, and then combined with crab meat, these skewers are definitely not something you can find at regular cookouts.

Ingredients:

- small tomato, chopped into bite-sized pieces
- ¼ cucumber, sliced
- crab stick, chopped into bite-sized pieces
- 3 black olives
- 2 lettuce leaves, chopped
- ½ cup of olive oil
- ¼ cup of fresh lime juice
- ½ tsp of sea salt

Preparation:

Shake together olive oil, fresh lime juice, and sea salt. Place the ingredients in this mixture and let it stand for about 3o minutes.

Place three wooden skewers into a large pot with some water to soak. This will prevent the skewers from burning. Remove the ingredients from the marinade and divide between the skewers. Grill for about 3-4 minutes, turning occasionally. Serve immediately.

20. Sweet Arugula Salad with Mixed Berry Dressing

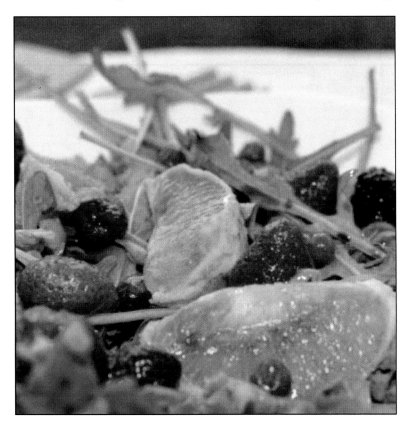

Arugula is a truly impressive green. Its nutty and slightly spicy flavor really pairs well with almost everything—fruits, vegetables, herbs, and spices. I always like to try something new. Fresh strawberries, tender raspberries, and blood orange soaked in sweet honey dressing will make you want more!

Ingredients (salad):

- 2 oz fresh arugula
- 1 orange, peeled and sectioned
- 5-6 fresh strawberries, sliced
- mixed berries
- ¼ cup of fresh cranberries

Ingredients (Berry Dressing):

- 1 tbsp of honey
- 3 tbsp of fresh lime juice
- 5 tbsp of fresh orange juice
- ¼ tsp of ground cinnamon

Preparation:

Whisk together 1 tablespoon of honey, fresh lime juice, orange juice, and ground cinnamon. Soak each piece of fruit into this mixture and transfer to a serving platter. Add fresh arugula and mix well. Serve cold.

21. Crispy Yellow Bean Salad with Lime Dressing

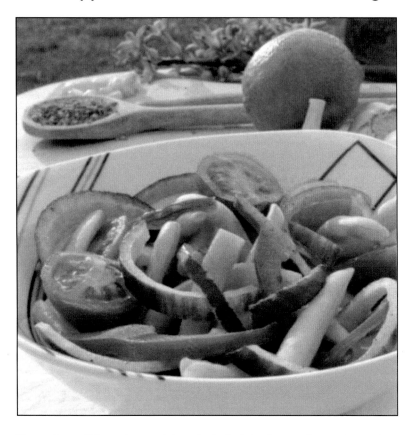

There is nothing about this salad that isn't excellent. From the fiber-rich and protein-packed yellow beans, to the lycopene loaded tomatoes, this salad shows off fresh spring taste in the best way. Make this salad ahead of time so the ingredients can marinade together for a more robust flavor.

Ingredients (salad):

- ½ red onion, peeled and sliced
- 1 cup of yellow beans, cooked
- 3 cherry tomatoes, halved
- 3 slices of red bell pepper

Ingredients (dressing):

- ¼ cup of fresh lime juice
- 3 tbsp of olive oil
- tsp of honey
- ½ small shallot, minced
- 1 garlic clove, crushed
- ¼ tsp of salt

Preparation:

Combine the lime juice with honey. Mix well with a fork. Slowly add the olive oil, whisking constantly. Now add the minced shallot, crushed garlic clove, and salt. Set aside.

Combine the ingredients in a medium-sized bowl. Add the dressing and toss well to combine. Serve cold.

22. Dandy Dandelion Salad

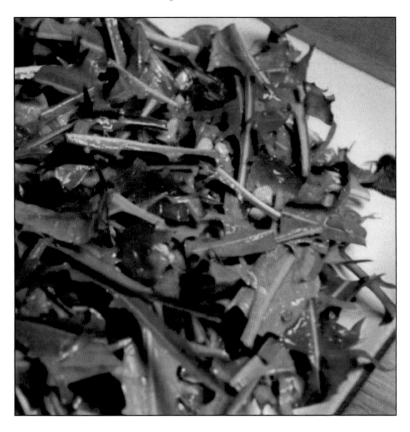

Yes, dandelion. The same plant that childhood memories of blowing puffy wishes are made of. The uniqueness of dandelion as a salad green should be enough to pique your interest. Delicate dandelion leaves provide a generous amount of vitamin C, fiber, potassium, iron, calcium, magnesium, zinc, and phosphorus, while almonds bring you healthy unsaturated fats. And the best part? Your husband won't believe that you're serving him the weed that he struggles to eradicate every spring from the front yard!

Ingredients:

- ½ pound of fresh dandelion greens, roughly chopped
- 1 small tomato, finely chopped
- ½ cup of Marcona almonds
- ½ cup of vegetable oil
- 1 tsp sherry vinegar
- Salt to taste

Preparation:

Roughly chop the dandelion greens and place in a bowl. Pour the oil over it and let it stand for about 3o minutes. Remove from the bowl and drain. Add finely chopped tomato and Marcona almonds. Season with salt and one teaspoon of sherry vinegar. Serve immediately.

23. Grilled Salmon over Spinach and Goat Cheese

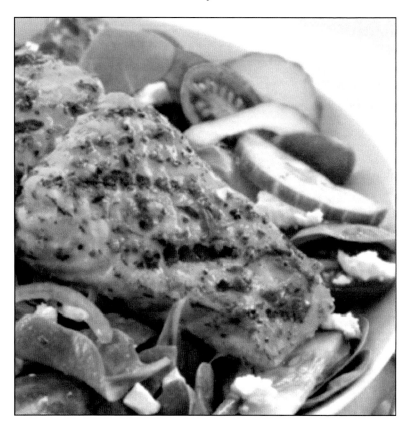

If you're looking for some new way of enjoying salmon, you've just found it! We all like this grilled fillet, but when combined with fresh goat cheese and vegetables, it becomes something a little naughty. I know what you're thinking. "Dr. Vuong! You can't have fish and cheese on the same dish!" Serving cheese with seafood is the new "bad boy" of cooking —everybody knows it's wrong, but they all want to find out how wrong for themselves.

Ingredients (salad):

- 3 oz salmon fillet, skin on preferred
- 1 cup of fresh spinach, roughly chopped
- 1/2 cucumber, sliced
- 5-6 cherry tomatoes
- 1 small red onion, sliced
- 1/2 cup of goat cheese
- salt and pepper

Ingredients (dressing):

- Extra virgin olive oil
- 1 tsp of dry rosemary, crushed
- 1 garlic clove, crushed
- Salt and pepper

Preparation:

Heat up some olive oil in a skillet, over medium-high temperature. Salt and pepper the salmon. After the oil is smoking, place the salmon fillet skin down, and fry for 5-6 minutes until the skin is crispy. Resist the urge to move the filet during that time. Flip the filet over for 2-3 minutes to bring to desired internal temperature. Remove from heat and use some kitchen paper towels to soak up any excess oil.

In a small bowl, combine ¼ cup of olive oil with one teaspoon of dry rosemary, crushed garlic, and some salt.

Place the salad ingredients in a large bowl and top with salmon. Drizzle with dressing. Serve.

24. Like Buttah Salad

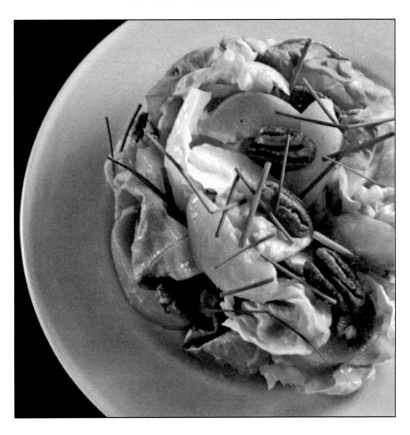

Butter lettuce has a crisp yet tender texture and a mildly sweet flavor, so it goes down easy. It's often interchanged with Boston and Bibb lettuce. But then you couldn't say, "Like buttah...." Grill the peaches to elevate the profile during a barbeque cookout. Add some orange juice for a little zing and transform this combination into an often talked-about starter dish.

Ingredients (salad):

- 1 head of butter lettuce, roughly chopped (you can substitute with Boston or Bibb lettuce)
- ½ medium-sized peach, peeled and sliced (grill for extra flavor)
- ½ cup of toasted pecan halves
- 2 snipped chives

Ingredients (dressing):

- ¼ cup of fresh orange juice
- 1 tbsp of honey
- ½ tsp of cinnamon

Preparation:

Whisk together the orange juice, honey, and cinnamon. Pour the orange mixture over lettuce and fruit. Arrange pecans on top and garnish with chives. Serve cold.

25. Watermelon Surprise Salad

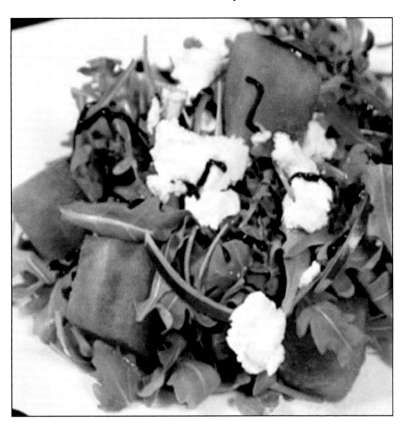

This unusual combination is the perfect way to use watermelon in a surprising way. Arugula with goat cheese is a classic combination, but once you add watermelon to this powder keg, the situation becomes explosive. A perfect, balsamic dressing will ignite this dish to life!

Ingredients (salad):

- 4 oz watermelon cubes
- ½ medium-sized red onion, sliced. (Soak rings in warm water to cut the bite.)
- A handful of fresh arugula
- ¼ cup of goat cheese, crumbled

Ingredients (dressing):

- 2 tbsp of balsamic vinegar
- 2 tbsp of extra virgin olive oil
- Salt and pepper to taste

Preparation:

Whisk together the dressing ingredients in a small bowl. Set aside.

Now combine the arugula and goat cheese with the watermelon cubes. Drizzle with balsamic vinegar dressing and serve.

26. Dinosaur Kale with Orange Sesame

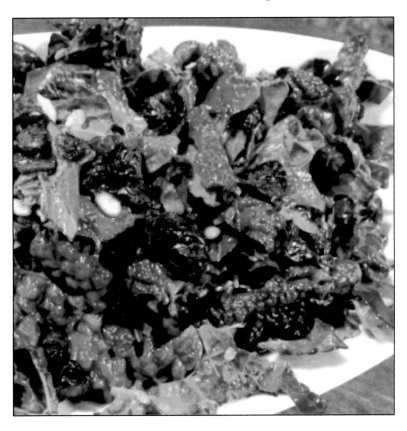

The lumpy bumpy texture of dinosaur kale and wrinkly skin of cranberries will remind you of something mesmerizing from Jurassic Park. But don't be scared. This salad is very approachable. With all of these vitamins, it's easy to see from where the Velociraptors got their strength.

Ingredients (salad):

- 1 bunch of dinosaur kale, roughly chopped
- ½ cup of dry cranberries
- pinon nuts (pine nuts)

Ingredients (dressing):

- ¼ cup of fresh orange juice
- 2 tbsp of toasted sesame oil
- tbsp of honey
- 2 tsp of ginger, minced

Preparation:

Combine fresh orange juice with toasted sesame oil, one tablespoon of honey, and minced ginger in a large bowl. Add cranberries and ginger. Toss to combine. Let it stand in the refrigerator for about 3o minutes.

Place dinosaur kale, cranberries, and pinon nuts in a large bowl and mix with orange dressing. Serve.

27. Quick Bean Salad

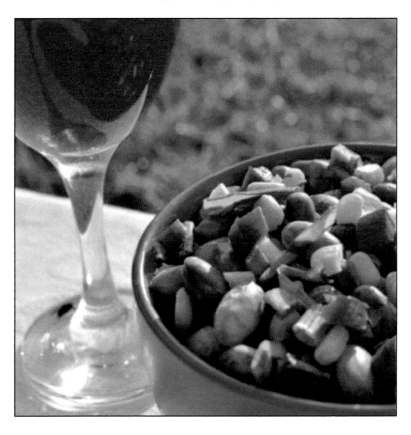

In a rush? Have leftover beans? Throw some into this salad bowl. Hot chili pepper is what gives this salad its kick, but don't stop there. Feel free to throw in some pickled jalapenos or porcini peppers.

Ingredients (salad):

- 1 cup of cooked beans
- ½ cup of sweet corn
- 3 spring onions, chopped
- ¼ small chili pepper, finely chopped

Ingredients (dressing):

- 3 tbsp of extra-virgin olive oil
- ½ tsp of red wine vinegar
- tsp of fresh lemon juice
- tsp of cilantro
- A pinch of salt

Preparation:

In a small bowl, combine the olive oil with red wine vinegar, fresh lemon juice, cilantro, and a pinch of salt. Mix well and use to season the other ingredients. Serve!

28. Caveman Chicken Salad

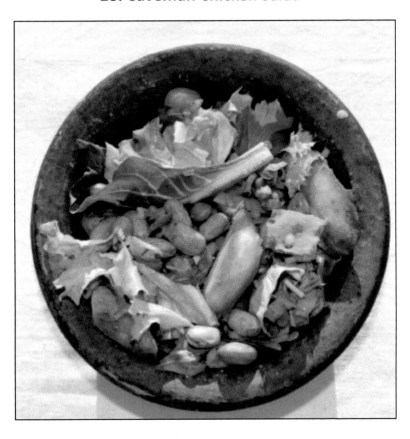

Created with lean protein from organic chicken and fresh lime juice, this recipe will create a perfect dinner for the hungry caveman and his cave-family. Simple ingredients. Robust flavor. No hunting involved.

Ingredients (salad):

- 1 piece of organic chicken breast, 0.5 inch thick, boneless and skinless
- olive oil
- salt and pepper
- cup of finely chopped butter lettuce
- Several spinach leaves
- ½ cup of cooked beans

Ingredients (dressing):

- 1 tbsp of fresh lime juice
- 1 tbsp of olive oil
- Pinch of salt

Preparation:

Add olive oil to a non-stick grill pan. Preheat over medium-high heat. Wash and pat dry the chicken. Salt and pepper each side. Cook for about 5-6 minutes on each side. Remove from the heat. Rest chicken for 10 minutes, then cut into several pieces.

Combine the meat with other ingredients, toss with vegetable oil, fresh lime juice, and a pinch of salt. Serve.

29. Green on Green Crime

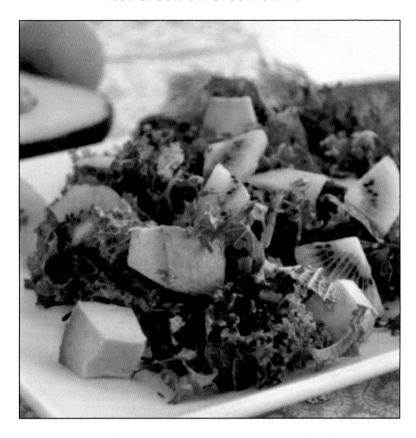

It's a travesty. Why can't we all just get along? Like Kermit said, "It's not easy being green." These green sisters learned to set their differences aside and elevate each other's games. After all, that's what friends are for...

Ingredients:

- bunch of kale, finely chopped
- ½ avocado, diced
- ¼ cup of fresh dill, chopped
- 1 kiwi, peeled and sliced
- 2 tbsp of olive oil
- ¼ cup of fresh lemon juice
- salt to taste

Preparation:

Wash and clean kale. Remove the stems. Place in a bowl. Add two tablespoons of olive oil and toss. Add dill, kiwi, avocado and fresh lemon juice. Salt to taste. Serve.

30. Dziugas Salad

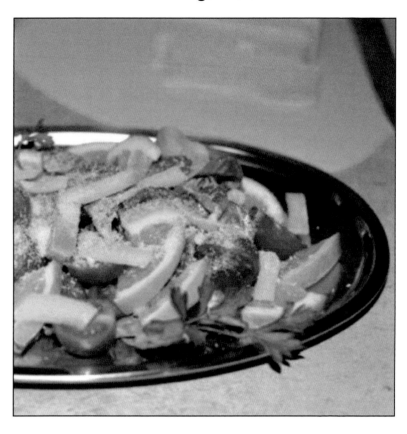

Legendary, hard fermented, Dziugas cheese comes from Lithuania. Its special, Parmesan-like flavor is the main reason Dziugas is an award winning cheese. This slightly eccentric combination of fresh orange slices and cherry tomatoes will brighten up your day. Try it and see for yourself why this cheese is so appreciated.

Ingredients:

- 1 cup of cherry tomatoes
- ½ cup of dziugas cheese, sliced (substitute with block parmesan)
- ½ cup of baby spinach
- 1 small orange
- 1 tbsp of Parmesan cheese
- Few parsley leaves
- 1 tsp of fresh lemon juice

Preparation:

Combine the ingredients in a large bowl and add lemon juice. Mix well and serve.

31. Purple Salad

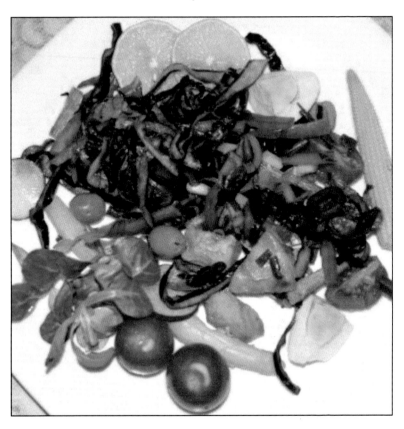

Purple cabbage is not just a healthy ingredient, but its intensive color makes it a beautiful addition on any plate. Served with other fresh vegetables, lean turkey meat, and hard boiled eggs can easily turn this salad into a lunch.

Ingredients:

- 1 piece of turkey breast, boneless and skinless
- 2 eggs
- 1 cup of red cabbage, grated
- 1 medium tomato
- ½ cup of olives
- cup of scallions, chopped
- Few artichoke hearts
- Few pieces of baby corn
- 2 tbsp of olive oil
- 2 tbsp of vegetable oil
- Salt to taste
- 1 tbsp of fresh lemon juice

Preparation:

Wash and pat dry the meat with a kitchen paper. Cut into 1 inch thick strips. In a large skillet, heat up the vegetable oil. Fry the turkey strips for about 10 minutes. Remove from the heat and soak the excess oil with a kitchen paper. Transfer to a large bowl.

Meanwhile boil the eggs for about 7-8 minutes. Remove from the heat, drain and peel. Cut into slices.

Add the remaining ingredients into the bowl and mix well. Season with some salt and fresh lemon juice.

Other Books by Dr. Duc Vuong

Meditate to Lose Weight: A Guide For A Slimmer Healthier You

Healthy Eating on a Budget: A How-To Guide

Eating Healthy for Kids: A How-To Guide

Healthy Green Smoothies: 50 Easy Recipes That Will Change Your Life

Big-Ass Salads: 31 Easy Recipes For Your Healthy Month

Weight Loss Surgery Success: Dr. V's A-Z Steps For Losing Weight And Gaining Enlightenment

The Ultimate Gastric Sleeve Success: A Practical Patient Guide

Lap-Band Rescue: Revisit. Rethink. Revise.

Duc-It-Up: 366 Tips To Improve Your Life

Made in the USA
Las Vegas, NV
17 November 2020